Hospice Palliative Care in Nepal

Workbook for Nurses

Katherine Murray

RN, BSN, MA, CHPCN(C)

Life and Death Matters

Saanichton BC

2013

Hospice Palliative Care in Nepal

Workbook for Nurses

by Katherine Murray

RN, BSN, MA, CHPCN(C)

Published by Life and Death Matters, 2958 Lamont Road, Saanichton, BC Canada, V8M 1W5
www.lifeanddeathmatters.ca

Editing and Production by Ann-Marie Gilbert
Design by Ann-Marie Gilbert.

Library and Archives Canada Cataloguing in Publication

Murray, Katherine, 1957-, author
Hospice palliative care in Nepal workbook : study guide
for nurses / Katherine Murray.

Companion to: Hospice palliative care in Nepal.
ISBN 978-1-926923-01-7 (pbk.)

1. Hospice care--Nepal--Handbooks, manuals, etc.
2. Palliative treatment--Nepal--Handbooks, manuals, etc.
3. Nursing--Nepal--Handbooks, manuals, etc. I. Title.

Disclaimer

This book is intended to be only a resource of general education on the subject matter. Every effort has been taken to ensure the accuracy of its information, however, there is no guarantee the information will remain current as time extends past the publication date. The information and techniques offered in this book should be used in consultation with qualified medical health professionals and should not be considered a replacement, substitute, or alternative for their guidance, assessment, or treatment. The author and publisher does not accept responsibility or liability to any person or entity with respect to loss or damage or any other problem caused or alleged to be caused directly or indirectly by information contained in this book

About the Cover

The arbutus tree, Canada's only native broadleaf evergreen, grows along the windblown Pacific coast, often on rock bluffs or in rocky soil. The Arbutus tree thrives where no others venture. This gnarled tree, with its eczema-like reddish-brown bark peeling off in papery flakes each spring, stands as a symbol of strength, commitment, perseverance, determination and survival, amidst so many adversities. In these ways, the Arbutus tree symbolizes the strength, beauty, and uniqueness of the human spirit and our ability to grow in the midst of suffering; and to live fully, even in the face of death and dying.

Christine Piercy writes, "The arbutus tree represents that place between life and death, often perched precariously at the meeting place of land and ocean. So it is with those who are dying and those who care for them, as the dying hover in this place of transition between life and death. Those of us who encircle them may long to bring them back into life, or wish that death would take them from this intensely painful place of 'in-between'. Is it possible that, like the Arbutus tree, there can be growth and beauty in such a place?"

Table of Contents

Introduction to Hospice Palliative Care

Define these terms:

1. Hospice: _____

_____

_____

2. Palliative Care:_____

_____

_____

3. A palliative approach: _____

_____

_____

4. Draw a diagram to illustrate the different individuals and groups of the health care team in your community.

5. Draw a diagram to illustrate the different participants and groups of the health care team in remote areas of your country.

6. List the names of the palliative care organizations in your country. _____

_____

_____

Standardized Assessment Tools

Provide full name and definitions for each of these words or terms.

7. PPS _____

_____

_____

8. ESAS _____

_____

_____

9. SAA _____

_____

_____

10. SBAR _____

_____

_____

11. Palliation _____

_____

_____

Provide short answers

12. List 8 common issues identified in the CHPCA Square of Care_____

_____

_____

_____

13. Describe the value of using standardized assessment tools _____

_____

_____

14. Describe the purpose of the PPS _____

_____

_____

15. List five symptoms that can be assessed using the ESAS tool? _____

_____

_____

16. Identify what the letters OPQRSTUV represent in the Symptom Assessment Acronym (SAA)

_____

_____

17. Identify at least three times when a symptom should be assessed _____

_____

18. List members of the health care team who can participate in assessment _____

_____

_____

19. What do the letters SBAR represent? How might this communication tool be useful? _____

_____

_____

Case Study #1

Ajay, a 65 year old male has primary cancer of the prostate and a recent diagnosis of metastasis to the bone. Ajay arrived on the unit where you work and you are assigned to care for him.

On the third day, Ajay is very slow to get out of bed. He holds his right hip and supports himself by holding on to furniture as he moves. This is very different from the last two days. Initially he denies there is any pain but does say he is "sore."

20. Form groups of three people to role play an assessment with Ajay. One person plays the part of Ajay, one person plays the nurse and the third person observes the role and makes notes to provide feedback to the performers. Rotate each person through each role, incorporating the feedback from each session into the next roleplay. Prepare to discuss your findings with the larger group. Use the space below for notes. _____

_____

_____

_____

_____

_____

_____

_____

21. Consider and discuss the following questions.

       a. When should pain be assessed?

       b. Who assesses pain?

       c. How can we identify pain without the patient saying he has pain?

       d. Discuss different types of pain.

       e. Identify comfort measures that may support someone in pain.

_____

_____

_____

_____

_____

_____

_____

_____

_____

_____

_____

_____

_____

_____

_____

_____

_____

_____

Symptom Management

Short answers

1. Identify five different routes for administering medications

   i _____

   ii. _____

   iii. _____

   iv. _____

   v. _____

Principles for Using Medications to Manage Symptoms

Define these terms.

2. Palliate/ Palliation _____

   _____

3. Titrate / Titration _____

   _____

4. Breakthrough doses _____

   _____

5. Adjuvant medications _____

   _____

6. List and briefly describe at least 6 principles for using medications to manage symptoms. _____

   _____

   _____

   _____

_____

_____

_____

_____

_____

_____

Using Opioids

1. Opioids are often useful in helping to manage _____ and _____ (two symptoms)

2. **True** or **False** The principles for titrating opioids can also be used when titrating other medications for managing other symptoms.

3. What opioids are available in your hospital? _____

_____

_____

_____

_____

4. List four common side effects of using opioids._____

_____

_____

_____

_____

5. List four fears of using opioids. _____

_____

_____

Equianalgesia Table for Opioids

Drug	Route Oral/ Rectal	Sub-cutaneous	Schedule
codeine	100mg	65mg	q4h
oxycodone	5.0 to 7.0 mg	-	q4h
morphine	10 mg	5 mg	q4h
hydromorphone	2 mg	1 mg	q4h
tramadol	1000 mg	-	-

Use a role play or large group discussion to demonstrate your understanding of the following concepts. Use the space provided below for notes for your role play or presentation or notes from other presentations.

6. Explain how you would teach a patient and family about the side effects of opioids.

_____

_____

_____

_____

_____

_____

_____

7. Explain ways to manage the side effects of opioid use. _____

_____

_____

_____

_____

_____

_____

8. Discuss concerns that family may express about addiction, tolerance, dependency. _____

_____

_____

_____

_____

_____

_____

_____

Calculating Opioid Doses

Calculations with Short Answers

9. Identify problems with the following analgesic orders

a. Morphine 10-15 mg *p.o. every 4-6 hours as needed* for severe pain.

_____

_____

b. Tylenol #3 1-2 *p.o. q6h prn* mild-moderate pain._____

_____

_____

c. Morphine 20 mg *p.o. q4h* and morphine 5 mg for breakthrough dose (BTD) as needed._____

_____

_____

10. Describe why opioids are given regularly, (*i.e.* every four hours) around the clock.

_____

_____

_____

Equianalgesia for Opioids

Note: It is not the role of the nurse to determine the exact dosage of opioid in conversions. Instead, the nurses role is to be familiar with the calculations and aware of appropriate dose ranges so that they will be able to help identify when a mistake is made in conversion, or to identify when the opioid order needs to be adjusted to better meet the needs of the patient.

Complete the following calculations.

11. A patient is currently taking codeine, 30 mgs *po*, 2 tabs *qid.*

   a. Calculate this patient's 24 hour dose of codeine._____

_____

_____

   b. Calculate this patient's 4 hour dose of codeine._____

_____

_____

_____

12. Calculate the equianalgesia dose of the following medications for this patient:

a. Morphine oral *q4h* - *?* mg dilaudid oral *q4h* _____

b. Morphine - long acting *q12h* = *?* mg dilaudid oral *q4h* _____

c. Morphine subcutaneous *q4h* = *?* mg dilaudid sc *q4h*_____

13. Calculate new medication doses for a patient currently taking **morphine 30mg *p.o. q4h***, wherein the physician has ordered a switch to hydromorphone.

a. Hydromorphone oral *q4h* _____

_____

b. Hydromorph long acting *p.o. q12h* _____

_____

c. Hydromorphone *s.c. q4h* _____

_____

Breakthrough Doses

14. What formulas is used in your area to determine breakthrough doses? _____

_____

_____

15. A physician is ordering morphine 10 mg *s.c. q4h.* What is an appropriate breakthrough dose? Why?

_____

_____

_____

16. The physician has ordered:
   • morphine 50 mg *p.o. q4h* and morphine 5 mg *p.o.* prn breakthrough dose.

a. Explain what is wrong with this breakthough dose. _____

_____

_____

_____

b. What is an appropriate breakthrough dose for this patient? _____

_____

_____

_____

17. Calculate the breakthrough dose for a patient receiving morphine long acting 60 mg *p.o. q12h?* __

_____

_____

18. Explain why more than one medication may be required to manage a symptom _____

_____

_____

19. List three routes for medication delivery _____ .

_____

_____

_____

Non Pharmacological Comfort Measures

1. Work with your classmates and develop a list of 25 things that you might do to offer comfort i.e. physical support, resources and psychosocial support.

_____

_____

_____

_____

_____

_____

_____

_____

_____

_____

_____

_____

_____

_____

_____

_____

_____

2. Demonstrate teaching a family caregiver various strategies for positioning a patient in bed for comfort, use pillows and blankets. (See *Appendix, Hospice Palliative Care in Nepal - A Resource for Nurses* for instructions).

3. Demonstrate teaching hand massage to a family caregiver.

Pain

1. Think of a time when you personally experienced pain. Was it a visceral pain like kidney stones or delivering a baby, a neuropathy like a burn, or a muscle bone pain like a broken bone. Which words did you use to describe the pain? What was helpful to you at the time? What was not helpful? ____

_____

_____

_____

_____

_____

2. Think of a patient who experienced pain that was not well managed. Write down what you can recall about the pain assessment and how the assessment was communicated to members of the health care team.

a. Were the patient and family involved in the assessment and planning of care? Explain why or why not.

_____

_____

_____

_____

_____

b. What pharmacological and nonpharmacological interventions were tried? _____

_____

_____

_____

Define these terms

3. Pain according to Margot McCaffery _____

_____

_____

_____

4. Total pain_____

_____

_____

5. What words might people use to describe a neuropathic type pain? _____

_____

6. What words might people use to describe a bone/muscle type pain?_____

_____

7. What words might people use to describe an visceral/organ pain?_____

_____

8. Explain five principles of pain management.' _____

_____

_____

_____

_____

_____

_____

_____

9. List five adjuvant medications used in pain management and how they contribute to pain management. _____

_____

_____

_____

_____

_____

Case Study #2

Work in groups of 3 individuals to answer all questions for the case study.

You have been assigned to care for Ahmed Bhatt, a 65 year old male with primary cancer of the prostate. He was recently diagnosed with metastatic bone cancer. Today he was admitted to the unit for pain and symptom management. Currently Ahmed received morphine 5 mg *po* every four hours at home and has not taken any breakthrough medication. Ahmed's wife is caring for him and she is very concerned.

In the emergency department morphine 5 mg *po q* 4-6 h *prn* was ordered, however no regular morphine was ordered.

You observe that Ahmed is very slow getting out of bed and often holds his right hip. He also supports himself by holding on to the bed as he moves. According to the patient chart, morphine 5mg *po* was given at 2200 and 0400. It is now 0730. No pain assessment has been completed. It is unclear where the pain is located and any other information about the pain. X-Rays are not available.

Role Play: Each person in the group plays one of the role play parts - patient, wife or nurse.

Complete a pain assessment using the SAA (Symptom Assessment Acronym).

As a team, document the assessment in the patient's chart.

Document and discuss concerns that team members have about the current orders.

_____

_____

_____

_____

_____

10. Use the SBAR to prepare a report for the physician.

11. Discuss the orders you expect the physician to give. _____

_____

_____

_____

Role Play:

Change the roles in the role play to: patient, doctor and an observer who will give feedback.

12. Using the SBAR, communicate the assessment, concerns, and recommendations to the doctor. Afterwards ask for feedback from the observer and adjust the communication accordingly. Work through the same SBAR communication again after changing roles, so that each person has the opportunity to work in each role. Incorporate feedback after each turn.

Feedback 1 _____

_____

Feedback 2 _____

_____

Feedback 3 _____

_____

13. Identify your own areas of difficulty in the communication process so that you can work on this on your own time. _____

_____

_____

_____

_____

14. As a team, discuss what steps would you take if you do not get orders that will help address Ahmed's pain? _____

_____

_____

Case Study #3

Work in groups of 3 individuals to answer all questions for the case study.

Ahmed and his wife are very anxious to have his pain controlled. At 10:30, the physician assesses Ahmed. and orders morphine 10mg *po* q4h and Morphine 5 mg *po prn* for breakthrough pain as needed.

On Day 2 Ahmed's pain is not yet controlled. According the patient chart he received morphine 10 mg *po q4h* as prescribed, and 3 breakthrough doses. He states that the regular dose does not take away his pain. He rates his current pain at 7/10. The physician suggests titrating the dose and adding in an adjuvant medication.

1. Calculate the new opioid dose using the two methods listed

    a. Method #1 - Increase according to the total daily dose _____

    _____

    _____

    _____

    b. Method #2 - Increase by percentage _____

    _____

    _____

    _____

2. The physician decided to give the morphine by subcutaneous route. Calculate the equivalent dose.

    _____

    _____

    _____

    _____

3. What adjuvants might be helpful? _____

    _____

    _____

Role play: Assume the roles of patient, nurse and wife.

The wife asks "Why does my husband need to be on so many medications?"

4. How would you respond to the wife? _____

_____

_____

_____

5. What are the most common side effects for someone receiving morphine and other opioids? ___

_____

_____

6. Think of what you might do proactively to prevent or identify side effects. _____

_____

_____

Case Study #4

Work in groups of 3 individuals to answer all questions for the case study.

You patient is Sabita Singh, a 79 year old woman with Alzheimer's Dementia, osteoarthritis and a fractured hip. She is not able to communicate verbally.

1. Discuss and compare the use of ESAS, SAA and PAIN AD when assessing someone with dementia.

_____

_____

_____

2. Discuss the unique issues of assessing pain when a patient has dementia. _____

_____

_____

_____

_____

_____

3. Discuss the importance of involving the family in assessment. _____

_____

_____

_____

_____

_____

Reflective question

4. Think back to the patient your wrote about whose pain was not well managed. How could
    the assessment and communication tools have assisted you in caring for this patient, and in
    communicating with the patient, family and members of the health care team? _____

_____

_____

_____

_____

5. What additional pharmacological and nonpharmacological interventions could have been helpful? _

_____

_____

_____

_____

Dyspnea

1. Think of a patient who was short of breath, and had difficulty breathing. Write in the space below any details that you recall about the assessment of their dyspnea and how their symptoms were communicated. _____

    _____

    _____

    _____

    _____

2. Were the patient and family involved in the assessment and planning of care? Explain._____

    _____

    _____

    _____

3. What pharmacological and nonpharmacological interventions were tried? _____

    _____

    _____

    _____

    _____

4. What words or phrases might trigger you to assess dyspnea? _____

    _____

    _____

    _____

5. Dyspnea cannot be assessed by objective measures alone. **True** or **False**

6. Oxygen is always helpful for someone who is dyspneic. **True** or **False**

7. List and briefly explain four principles for using medications to manage dyspnea. _____

_____

_____

_____

_____

_____

_____

_____

_____

Case Study#5

Work in groups of 3 individuals to answer all questions for the case study.

Santosh is 52 years old, and presents with cancer of the esophagus that has spread to the liver. Santosh is very short of breath. He rates his breathing discomfort at 7/10 and appears anxious. At home he received a benzodiazepine and bronchodilators via nebulizer. He states that these medications did not decrease his shortness of breath. Santosh has just arrived on your unit and the physician has not seen him. There are no orders for medication.

8. Describe ways that you would adapt the SAA to assess dyspnea. What questions would you ask? _

_____

_____

_____

_____

_____

_____

_____

9. What additional observations might you make that would be helpful in completing your assessment?

_____

_____

_____

_____

_____

_____

Role play

Work in groups of three, with each person assuming a role - patient, family member or nurse.

10. Role play through a dyspnea assessment using the SAA (Symptom Assessment Acronym).

11. Working as a team, document the assessment in the patient's chart.

12. Use the SBAR to help you prepare a report for the physician.

13. Discuss what type of orders you would expect the physician to give._____

_____

_____

_____

_____

_____

14. Change the roles to: patient, doctor and an observer who will give feedback. Use the SBAR to communicate the assessment, concerns, and recommendations to the doctor. Each person takes a turn at each role, incorporating the feedback from the previous roleplay.

Feedback 1 _____

_____

_____

Feedback 2 _____

_____

_____

Feedback 3 _____

_____

_____

Case Study #6

The physician orders morphine 2.5 mg *po q4h* and Morphine *1.25 mg po prn* for breakthrough dyspnea. The daughter is concerned and asks "What is dyspnea?" and "How will morphine help him breath better?" "Can he have oxygen?"

Role play: Each person takes one role - patient, family member or nurse.

1. Teach the daughter about dyspnea, and why morphine is helpful for dyspnea, and explore the benefits

_____

_____

_____

2. Working as a team, review the process for titrating opioids for a person with dyspnea. _____

_____

_____

_____

3. Identify nonpharmacological comfort measures for someone with dyspnea._____

_____

_____

_____

_____

4. Why is it important to remain calm? _____

_____

_____

Role play: Rotate through playing the patient, nurse and observer.

5. Santosh becomes very dyspneic. Coach Santosh when he is short of breath. _____

_____

_____

_____

_____

Case Study #7

Nadia is 79 years old with end-stage cardiac disease and chronic obstructive pulmonary disease. She has declined rapidly over the past two weeks, showing increased fatigue and decreased strength. Nadia is now unable to get out of bed. She was using a bed pan but was very short of breath when moving. Therefore she is now wearing an incontinence pad. Nadia has experienced periods of confusion in the past few days, is less alert and her only intake has been fluids over the last 48 hours.

Nadia experienced a sudden increased difficulty with breathing during the night. Shortness of breath increases with any attempt to talk. She is unable to rate her dyspnea. Her respirations are moist sounding.

Observations - Edema +3 legs up to her knees. Uses intercoastal muscles for breathing. Gasping for breath on admission. Unable to rate her dyspnea. Weak productive cough. Respiratory rate 30/min. Skin cool, clammy, diaphoretic.

Work in groups of 3 individuals to answer all questions for the case study.

1. Discuss comfort measures that might be helpful to implement immediately._____

_____

_____

_____

_____

_____

2. Family ask for oxygen to be started. You give oxygen via a mask. Nadia becomes more anxious and tries to pull the oxygen off. The family ask if suctioning the secretions would be helpful. What is your response? _____

_____

_____

_____

_____

3. What medications might be helpful and why? _____

_____

_____

_____

_____

_____

_____

_____

4. Could Nadia be dying? (Refer to the chapter on dying with chronic illness.) _____

_____

_____

_____

5. What are the challenges of prognosticating for Nadia? _____

_____

_____

_____

6. Describe causes of pre-death respiratory congestion._____

_____

_____

_____

_____

_____

7. List common medications to control respiratory congestion. _____

_____

_____

_____

8. Describe nonpharmacological comfort measures for respiratory congestion. _____

_____

_____

_____

_____

_____

Role play: Work in groups of three, playing the family member, the nurse and the observer (to give feedback at the end).

9. Explain to the family about respiratory congestion, causes, and comfort measures._____

_____

_____

_____

_____

_____

10. Think back to the patient you reflected on earlier. How could the assessment and communication tools have assisted you in caring for this patient, and in communicating with the patient, family and members of the health care team? _____

_____

_____

_____

_____

_____

11. What additional pharmacological and nonpharmacological interventions could have been helpful? _

_____

_____

_____

_____

_____

_____

_____

Nausea and Vomiting

1. Think of a patient who was nauseated and vomiting. Describe the symptom assessment, how the assessment was communicated to the health care team and the care provided. _____

_____

_____

_____

2. Was the patient and family involved in the assessment and planning of care? _____

_____

_____

3. What pharmacological and nonpharmacological interventions were tried? _____

_____

_____

_____

4. Use the body map to identify and label causes of nausea and vomiting.

Please mark on these pictures where it is you hurt.

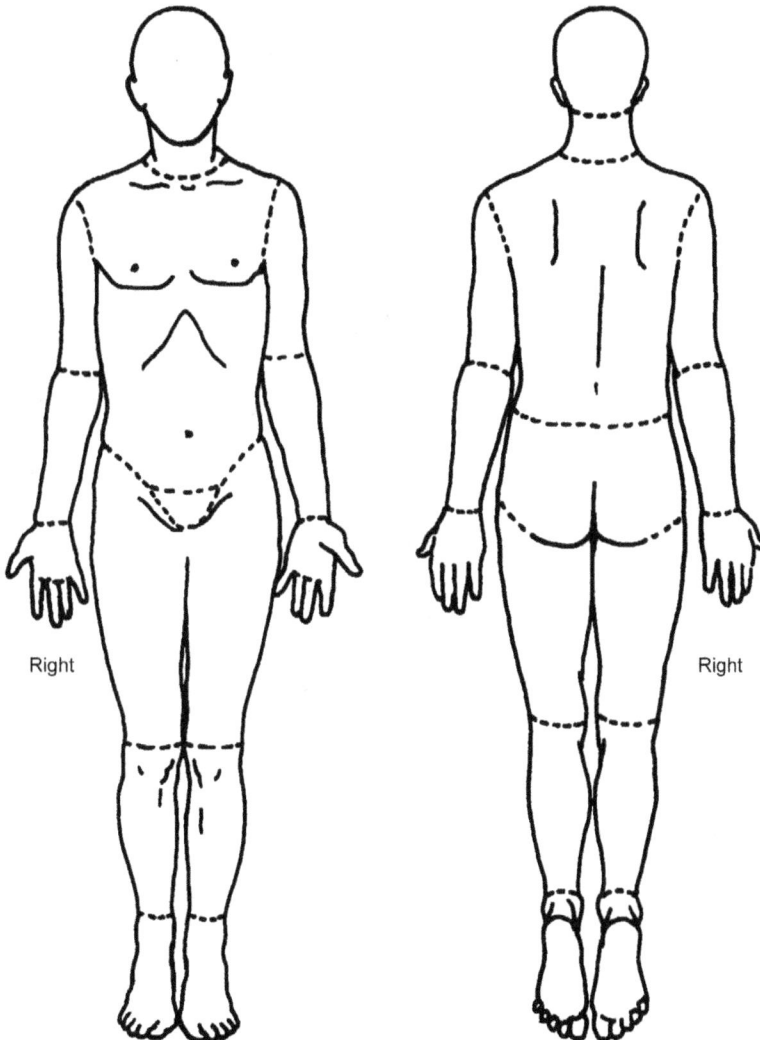

Right   Right

5. Explain why different types of medications may be needed to palliate nausea and vomiting. _____

_____

_____

_____

_____

_____

_____

6. In this list below, link the cause of nausea with one of the most appropriate medications to help decrease the nausea and vomiting.

Haldol or Nozinan	bowel obstruction caused by tumour pressing on intestines
Gravol	constipation
Dexamethasone	vomiting partially digested food
Maxeran	started on opioid and immediately vomited
Sennokot	motion sickness

7. List and explain principles used when managing nausea and vomiting._____

_____

_____

_____

_____

_____

_____

Case Study #8

Sabita, a 54 year old woman, has cancer of the tongue and an infection of the jaw bone. She was admitted because of pain and started on morphine 5 mg *po q4h* at 1000 this morning. She was nauseated at 1200, and vomited the 1400 dose. No prior history of nausea, and no prior experience with morphine. Was on Tramadol at home.

Work together as a team of three to answer these questions.

1. What are the possible causes of nausea and vomiting? _____

   _____

   _____

   _____

2. Adapt the questions from SAA to assess nausea and vomiting._____

   _____

   _____

   _____

   _____

   _____

   _____

   _____

   _____

3. What additional assessment and observations might you want to complete? _____

   _____

   _____

   _____

   _____

4. Complete an assessment of the nausea and vomiting using the SAA.

5. Document the assessment in the patients chart.

6. Use the SBAR to help you prepare a report for the physician.

7. Discuss what type of orders you would expect the physician to give._____

_____

_____

_____

_____

Role Play - Work again in the same group of three, this time one person will be the patient, one the doctor, and the other will observe and give feedback.

8. Use the SBAR to communicate the assessment, concerns, and recommendations to the doctor.

_____

_____

Case Study #9

1. The physician's orders for Sabita are:

   - Morphine 2.5 mg sc *q4h*, with Morphine 1.25 *mg* sc for breakthrough symptom *prn*
   - Halperidol 1 mg sc *bid*
   - Antibiotic IV

Working together as a team, answer the following questions.

2. Discuss nonpharmacological comfort measures for managing nausea and supporting a person who is vomiting. _____

_____

_____

_____

_____

_____

_____

_____

3. Think back to the patient you reflected on earlier. How could the assessment and communication tools have assisted you in caring for this patient, and in communicating with the patient, family and members of the health care team? Explain._____

_____

_____

_____

_____

_____

Cachexia and Anorexia

1. Think about how you have felt when a loved on or patient stopped eating. Write briefly about this experience. _____

_____

_____

_____

_____

Define

2. Cachexia _____

_____

_____

3. Anorexia _____

_____

_____

Case Study #10

Anchita is a 64 year old grandmother with lung cancer and was admitted two weeks ago to the unit. At home she was declining steadily over the past months, suffering repeated chest infections. According to family she shows increasing weakness and falls if she is not assisted.

Since her admission to the unit, she is sleeping longer and more frequently, is refusing food and shows some difficulty swallowing. Anchita's son cares for her during the day and sleeps at her bedside at night.

Today her daughter arrived and is very concerned that if Anchita does not eat more that she will get sick and die. She is alarmed by her mother's weight loss and came to you to say that her mother is "starving." She believes that decreased nutritional intake is responsible for her declining condition.

Working in a small group as a team and address the following questions:

4. What are the characteristics that define anorexia and cachexia? _____

_____

_____

_____

_____

_____

_____

5. What causes anorexia and cachexia? _____

_____

_____

_____

_____

_____

6. Do anorexia and cachexia always happen together? _____

_____

_____

_____

_____

7. Is this the same as starvation? _____

_____

_____

Role play: One person playing the role of the nurse, a second person playing the family member and the third person observing and providing feedback to the role play members.

8. Family member asks "Will she die because she is not eating?" _____

_____

_____

_____

_____

9. Family member asks "Will she be hungry?" _____

_____

_____

_____

10. Family member asks "What can we do to keep her comfortable?" _____

_____

_____

_____

_____

Oral Discomfort

Work together in a small group team to answer these questions.

1. Revise the SAA questions to assess oral discomfort. Which questions seem particularly applicable? Are there any questions that are not useful? _____

_____

_____

_____

_____

_____

2. List common causes of oral discomfort? _____

_____

_____

_____

_____

3. What does thrush look like? _____

_____

_____

4. Why is thrush a common infection in the dying?_____

_____

_____

_____

5. What medications might be ordered for oral thrush? _____

_____

_____

6. What nonpharmacological comfort measures can you integrate?_____

_____

_____

_____

Dehydration

1. Why is dehydration a normal change for many people in the last few days. _____

_____

_____

_____

2. Discuss the advantages and disadvantages of artificial hydration in the last days of life. _____

_____

_____

_____

3. Identify situations when it might be appropriate to treat dehydration through artificial hydration. _

_____

_____

_____

_____

4. Identify situations when it might be inappropriate to treat dehydration through artificial hydration.

_____

_____

_____

_____

_____

5. Describe ways the family can nurture the patient without providing artificial hydration. _____

_____

_____

_____

_____

Delirium

Define

1. Delirium _____

_____

_____

_____

Reflective Exercise

2. Compare and contrast delirium, dementia and depression. _____

_____

_____

_____

3. List the causes of delirium. _____

_____

_____

_____

4. Which of these causes are normal changes in the dying process?_____

_____

_____

_____

_____

5. What are five characteristics of delirium? _____

_____

_____

_____

_____

6. Is delirium reversible?_____

_____

_____

_____

_____

7. What is terminal delirium? _____

_____

_____

_____

8. What is the pharmacological approach to managing delirium in palliative care?_____

_____

_____

_____

_____

_____

9. When might it be appropriate to attempt to reverse delirium? _____

_____

_____

_____

_____

_____

10. When might it not be appropriate to attempt to review delirium?_____

_____

_____

_____

_____

11. What might the family do to provide comfort?_____

_____

_____

_____

Constipation

1. What are the common causes of constipation in the palliative care patient? _____

_____

_____

_____

_____

_____

2. What comfort strategies might be useful to prevent and/or treat constipation? _____

_____

_____

_____

_____

_____

Diarrhea

1. What are the common causes of diarrhea in the palliative care patient? _____

_____

_____

_____

2. What comfort strategies might be useful to prevent and/or treat diarrhea? _____

_____

_____

_____

Pre-Death Restlessness

1. What is pre-death or terminal restlessness?_____

   _____

   _____

   _____

2. What comfort strategies might be useful in caring for the patient with pre-death restlessness? ____

   _____

   _____

   _____

3. What comfort strategies might be useful in supporting the family? _____

   _____

   _____

   _____

Pre-Death Awareness and Symbolic Communication

1. What is pre-death awareness? How would you support the patient and the family?_____

   _____

   _____

   _____

2. What is symbolic communication? How would you support the patient and the family? _____

   _____

   _____

   _____

SUPPORT FOR THE LAST DAYS AND HOURS

1. Families may ask when will death occur? Discuss in your group how you might respond to this question. _____

_____

_____

_____

_____

_____

2. Why is it especially challenging to answer this question when people are dying with chronic illness?

_____

_____

_____

_____

_____

3. List five sentinel events that might indicate that a person with late stage dementia is dying._____

_____

_____

4. Could these sentinel events be similar for people dying with other chronic illnesses? Please explain your answer. _____

_____

_____

_____

_____

5. Discuss how reviewing with the family the patients condition over the past months, weeks and days can help family and health care team understand the declining condition and when death may occur.

_____

_____

_____

_____

_____

_____

Psychosocial Implications of Physical Changes

For each of the physical changes that may occur in the last days and hours, identify i)one psychosocial implication for the family, and ii) one comfort measure for the patient.

1. Increased drowsiness - i) _____

_____

   ii) _____

_____

2. Reduced intake - i)_____

_____

   ii) _____

_____

3. Confusion and restlessness - i) _____

_____

   ii) _____

_____

4. Difficulty swallowing - i) _____

_____

   ii) _____

_____

5. Unresponsiveness - i) _____

_____

   ii) _____

_____

6. Changes in breathing sounds - i) _____

_____

   ii) _____

_____

7. Changes in skin colour and temperature - i) _____

_____

   ii) _____

_____

8. Twitching - i) _____

_____

   ii) _____

_____

9. Eyes, open or closed - i) _____

_____

   ii) _____

10. Bowel and bladder - i) _____

_____

ii) _____

_____

11. Breathing and expression at time of death - i) _____

_____

ii) _____

_____

12. You are assigned to pronounce death. What physical assessment needs to be completed? _____

_____

_____

_____

_____

13. Who needs to be notified? _____

_____

_____

_____

14. What needs to be documented after death? _____

_____

_____

_____

_____

Care of the Body

Discuss as a team:

1. Who is involved in the care of the body following death? _____

_____

_____

_____

_____

2. What is the responsibility of the different team members? _____

_____

_____

_____

_____

3. What is the nurse's responsibility?_____

_____

_____

_____

_____

4. What family and or cultural rituals are done following death? _____

_____

_____

_____

_____

5. What is the hospital or community policy for pronouncing and registering a death in your area?___

_____

_____

_____

_____

_____

www.ingramcontent.com/pod-product-compliance
Lightning Source LLC
Chambersburg PA
CBHW082113210326
41599CB00033B/6693